YOUR GUIDE TO
Lowering Your Blood Pressure With DASH

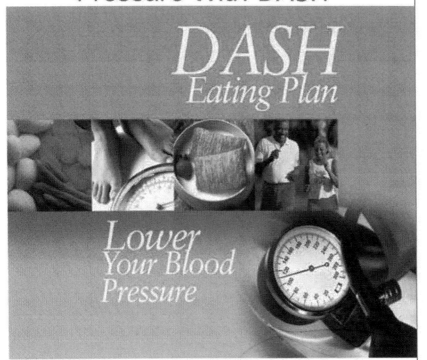

DASH
Eating Plan

Lower
Your Blood
Pressure

U.S. DEPARTMENT OF HEALTH AND HUMAN SERVICES
National Institutes of Health
National Heart, Lung, and Blood Institute

NIH Publication No. 06-4082
Originally Printed 1998
Revised April 2006

Contents

Introduction 1

What Is High Blood Pressure? 3

What Is the DASH Eating Plan? 5
    How Do I Make the DASH? 7
    How Can I Get Started on the DASH Eating Plan? 23

A Week With the DASH Eating Plan 29

Recipes for Heart Health 45

To Learn More 55

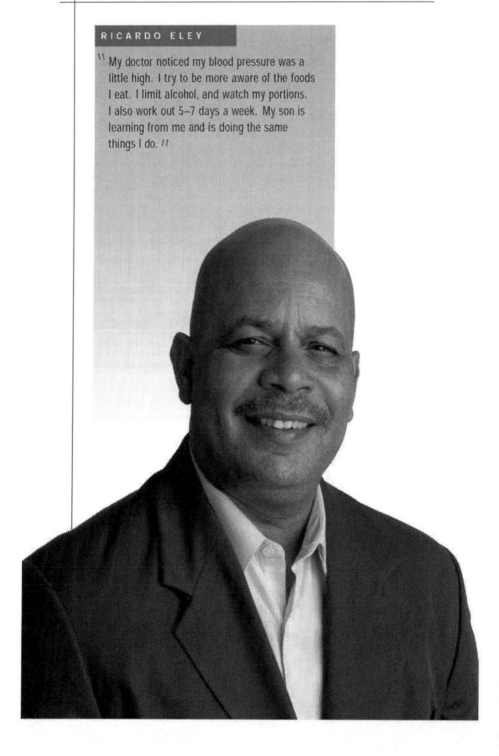

"My doctor noticed my blood pressure was a little high. I try to be more aware of the foods I eat. I limit alcohol, and watch my portions. I also work out 5–7 days a week. My son is learning from me and is doing the same things I do."

Introduction

What you choose to eat affects your chances of developing high blood pressure, or hypertension (the medical term). Recent studies show that blood pressure can be lowered by following the Dietary Approaches to Stop Hypertension (DASH) eating plan—and by eating less salt, also called sodium.

While each step alone lowers blood pressure, the combination of the eating plan and a reduced sodium intake gives the biggest benefit and may help prevent the development of high blood pressure.

This booklet, based on the DASH research findings, tells how to follow the DASH eating plan and reduce the amount of sodium you consume. It offers tips on how to start and stay on the eating plan, as well as a week of menus and some recipes. The menus and recipes are given for two levels of daily sodium consumption— 2,300 and 1,500 milligrams per day. Twenty-three hundred milligrams is the highest level considered acceptable by the National High Blood Pressure Education Program. It is also the highest amount recommended for healthy Americans by the 2005 "U.S. Dietary Guidelines for Americans." The 1,500 milligram level can lower blood pressure further and more recently is the amount recommended by the Institute of Medicine as an adequate intake level and one that most people should try to achieve.

The lower your salt intake is, the lower your blood pressure. Studies have found that the DASH menus containing 2,300 milligrams of sodium can lower blood pressure and that an even lower level of sodium, 1,500 milligrams, can further reduce blood pressure. All the menus are lower in sodium than what adults in the United States currently eat—about 4,200 milligrams per day in men and 3,300 milligrams per day in women.

Those with high blood pressure and prehypertension may benefit especially from following the DASH eating plan and reducing their sodium intake.

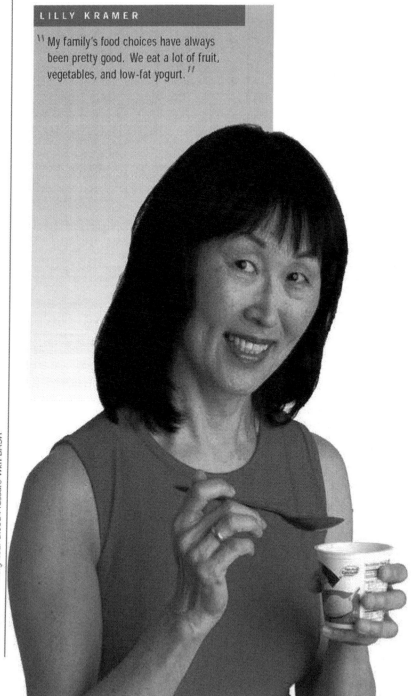

LILLY KRAMER

" My family's food choices have always been pretty good. We eat a lot of fruit, vegetables, and low-fat yogurt. "

What Is High Blood Pressure?

Blood pressure is the force of blood against artery walls. It is measured in millimeters of mercury (mmHg) and recorded as two numbers—systolic pressure (when the heart beats) over diastolic pressure (when the heart relaxes between beats). Both numbers are important. (See box 1 on page 4.)

Blood pressure rises and falls during the day. But when it stays elevated over time, then it's called high blood pressure. High blood pressure is dangerous because it makes the heart work too hard, and the high force of the blood flow can harm arteries and organs such as the heart, kidneys, brain, and eyes. High blood pressure often has no warning signs or symptoms. Once it occurs, it usually lasts a lifetime. If uncontrolled, it can lead to heart and kidney disease, stroke, and blindness.

High blood pressure affects more than 65 million—or 1 in 3—American adults. About 28 percent of American adults ages 18 and older, or about 59 million people, have prehypertension, a condition that also increases the chance of heart disease and stroke. High blood pressure is especially common among African Americans, who tend to develop it at an earlier age and more often than Whites. It is also common among older Americans—individuals with normal blood pressure at age 55 have a 90 percent lifetime risk for developing high blood pressure.

High blood pressure can be controlled if you take these steps:

- Maintain a healthy weight.
- Be moderately physically active on most days of the week.
- Follow a healthy eating plan, which includes foods lower in sodium.
- If you drink alcoholic beverages, do so in moderation.
- If you have high blood pressure and are prescribed medication, take it as directed.

All steps but the last also help to prevent high blood pressure.

BOX 1

Blood Pressure Levels for Adults*

Category	Systolic† (mmHg)‡		Diastolic† (mmHg)‡	Result
Normal	Less than 120	and	Less than 80	Good for you!
Prehypertension	120–139	or	80–89	Your blood pressure could be a problem. Make changes in what you eat and drink, be physically active, and lose extra weight. If you also have diabetes, see your doctor.
Hypertension	140 or higher	or	90 or higher	You have high blood pressure. Ask your doctor or nurse how to control it.

* For adults ages 18 and older who are not on medicine for high blood pressure and do not have a short-term serious illness. Source: The Seventh Report of the Joint National Committee on Prevention, Detection, Evaluation, and Treatment of High Blood Pressure; NIH Publication No. 03-5230, National High Blood Pressure Education Program, May 2003.

† If systolic and diastolic pressures fall into different categories, overall status is the higher category.

‡ Millimeters of mercury.

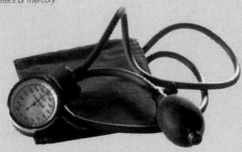

What Is the DASH Eating Plan?

Blood pressure can be unhealthy even if it stays only slightly above the normal level of less than 120/80 mmHg. The more your blood pressure rises above normal, the greater the health risk.

Scientists supported by the National Heart, Lung, and Blood Institute (NHLBI) conducted two key studies. Their findings showed that blood pressures were reduced with an eating plan that is low in saturated fat, cholesterol, and total fat and that emphasizes fruits, vegetables, and fat-free or low-fat milk and milk products. This eating plan—known as the DASH eating plan—also includes whole grain products, fish, poultry, and nuts. It is reduced in lean red meat, sweets, added sugars, and sugar-containing beverages compared to the typical American diet. It is rich in potassium, magnesium, and calcium, as well as protein and fiber. (See box 2 for the DASH studies' daily nutrient goals.)

BOX 2

Daily Nutrient Goals Used in the DASH Studies
(for a 2,100 Calorie Eating Plan)

Total fat	27% of calories	Sodium	2,300 mg*
Saturated fat	6% of calories	Potassium	4,700 mg
Protein	18% of calories	Calcium	1,250 mg
Carbohydrate	55% of calories	Magnesium	500 mg
Cholesterol	150 mg	Fiber	30 g

* 1,500 mg sodium was a lower goal tested and found to be even better for lowering blood pressure. It was particularly effective for middle-aged and older individuals, African Americans, and those who already had high blood pressure.
g = grams; mg = milligrams

The DASH eating plan follows heart healthy guidelines to limit saturated fat and cholesterol. It focuses on increasing intake of foods rich in nutrients that are expected to lower blood pressure, mainly minerals (like potassium, calcium, and magnesium), protein, and fiber. It includes nutrient-rich foods so that it meets other nutrient requirements as recommended by the Institute of Medicine.

The first DASH study involved 459 adults with systolic blood pressures of less than 160 mmHg and diastolic pressures of 80–95 mmHg. About 27 percent of the participants had high blood pressure. About 50 percent were women and 60 percent were African Americans. It compared three eating plans: a plan that includes foods similar to what many Americans regularly eat; a plan that includes foods similar to what many Americans regularly eat plus more fruits and vegetables; and the DASH eating plan. All three plans included about 3,000 milligrams of sodium daily. None of the plans was vegetarian or used specialty foods.

Results were dramatic. Participants who followed both the plan that included more fruits and vegetables and the DASH eating plan had reduced blood pressure. But the DASH eating plan had the

Who Helped With DASH?

The DASH studies were sponsored by the NHLBI and conducted at four medical centers. There was also a central coordinating center at Kaiser Permanente Center for Health Research in Portland, OR. The four medical centers were: Brigham and Women's Hospital, Boston, MA; Duke Hypertension Center and the Sarah W. Stedman Nutrition and Metabolism Center, Durham, NC; Johns Hopkins Medical Institutions, Baltimore, MD; and Pennington Biomedical Research Center, Baton Rouge, LA.

greatest effect, especially for those with high blood pressure. Furthermore, the blood pressure reductions came fast—within 2 weeks of starting the plan.

The second DASH study looked at the effect on blood pressure of a reduced dietary sodium intake as participants followed either the DASH eating plan or an eating plan typical of what many Americans consume. This second study involved 412 participants. Participants were randomly assigned to one of the two eating plans and then followed for a month at each of the three sodium levels. The three sodium levels were a higher intake of about 3,300 milligrams per day (the level consumed by many Americans), an intermediate intake of about 2,300 milligrams per day, and a lower intake of about 1,500 milligrams per day.

Results showed that reducing dietary sodium lowered blood pressure for both eating plans. At each sodium level, blood pressure was lower on the DASH eating plan than on the other eating plan. The greatest blood pressure reductions were for the DASH eating plan at the sodium intake of 1,500 milligrams per day. Those with high blood pressure saw the greatest reductions, but those with prehypertension also had large decreases.

Together these studies show the importance of lowering sodium intake—whatever your eating plan. For a true winning combination, follow the DASH eating plan and lower your intake of salt and sodium.

How Do I Make the DASH?

The DASH eating plan used in the studies calls for a certain number of daily servings from various food groups. These are given in box 3 on page 8 for 2,000 calories per day. The number of servings you require may vary, depending on your caloric need. Box 4 on page 10 gives the number of servings for 1,600, 2,600, and 3,100 calories.

The DASH eating plan used along with other lifestyle changes can help you prevent and control blood pressure. If your blood pressure is not too high, you may be able to control it entirely by changing your eating habits, losing weight if you are overweight, getting regular physical activity, and cutting down on alcohol. The DASH eating plan also has other benefits, such as lowering LDL ("bad") cholesterol, which, along with lowering blood pressure, can reduce your risk for getting heart disease.

BOX 3

Following the DASH Eating Plan

Food Group	Daily Servings	Serving Sizes
Grains*	6–8	1 slice bread 1 oz dry cereal† 1/2 cup cooked rice, pasta, or cereal
Vegetables	4–5	1 cup raw leafy vegetable 1/2 cup cut-up raw or cooked vegetable 1/2 cup vegetable juice
Fruits	4–5	1 medium fruit 1/4 cup dried fruit 1/2 cup fresh, frozen, or canned fruit 1/2 cup fruit juice
Fat-free or low-fat milk and milk products	2–3	1 cup milk or yogurt 11/2 oz cheese
Lean meats, poultry, and fish	6 or less	1 oz cooked meats, poultry, or fish 1 egg‡
Nuts, seeds, and legumes	4–5 per week	1/3 cup or 11/2 oz nuts 2 Tbsp peanut butter 2 Tbsp or 1/2 oz seeds 1/2 cup cooked legumes (dry beans and peas)
Fats and oils§	2–3	1 tsp soft margarine 1 tsp vegetable oil 1 Tbsp mayonnaise 2 Tbsp salad dressing
Sweets and added sugars	5 or less per week	1 Tbsp sugar 1 Tbsp jelly or jam 1/2 cup sorbet, gelatin 1 cup lemonade

* Whole grains are recommended for most grain servings as a good source of fiber and nutrients.

† Serving sizes vary between 1/2 cup and 11/4 cups, depending on cereal type. Check the product's Nutrition Facts label.

The DASH eating plan shown below is based on 2,000 calories a day. The number of daily servings in a food group may vary from those listed depending on your caloric needs. Use this chart to help you plan your menus or take it with you when you go to the store.

Examples and Notes	Significance of Each Food Group to the DASH Eating Pattern
Whole wheat bread and rolls, whole wheat pasta, English muffin, pita bread, bagel, cereals, grits, oatmeal, brown rice, unsalted pretzels and popcorn	Major sources of energy and fiber
Broccoli, carrots, collards, green beans, green peas, kale, lima beans, potatoes, spinach, squash, sweet potatoes, tomatoes	Rich sources of potassium, magnesium, and fiber
Apples, apricots, bananas, dates, grapes, oranges, grapefruit, grapefruit juice, mangoes, melons, peaches, pineapples, raisins, strawberries, tangerines	Important sources of potassium, magnesium, and fiber
Fat-free (skim) or low-fat (1%) milk or butter-milk, fat-free, low-fat, or reduced-fat cheese, fat-free or low-fat regular or frozen yogurt	Major sources of calcium and protein
Select only lean; trim away visible fats; broil, roast, or poach; remove skin from poultry	Rich sources of protein and magnesium
Almonds, hazelnuts, mixed nuts, peanuts, walnuts, sunflower seeds, peanut butter, kidney beans, lentils, split peas	Rich sources of energy, magnesium, protein, and fiber
Soft margarine, vegetable oil (such as canola, corn, olive, or safflower), low-fat mayon-naise, light salad dressing	The DASH study had 27 per-cent of calories as fat, including fat in or added to foods
Fruit-flavored gelatin, fruit punch, hard candy, jelly, maple syrup, sorbet and ices, sugar	Sweets should be low in fat

† Since eggs are high in cholesterol, limit egg yolk intake to no more than four per week; two egg whites have the same protein content as 1 oz of meat.

§ Fat content changes serving amount for fats and oils. For example, 1 Tbsp of regular salad dressing equals one serving; 1 Tbsp of a low-fat dressing equals one-half serving; 1 Tbsp of a fat-free dressing equals zero servings.

BOX 4

DASH Eating Plan— Number of Daily Servings for Other Calorie Levels

	Servings/Day		
Food Groups	1,600 calories/day	2,600 calories/day	3,100 calories/day
Grains*	6	10–11	12–13
Vegetables	3–4	5–6	6
Fruits	4	5–6	6
Fat-free or low-fat milk and milk products	2–3	3	3–4
Lean meats, poultry, and fish	3–6	6	6–9
Nuts, seeds, and legumes	3/week	1	1
Fats and oils	2	3	4
Sweets and added sugars	0	≤2	≤2

* *Whole grains are recommended for most grain servings as a good source of fiber and nutrients.*

If you need to lose weight, even a small weight loss will help to lower your risks of developing high blood pressure and other serious health conditions. At the very least, you should not gain weight. A recent study showed that people can lose weight while following the DASH eating plan and lowering their sodium intake. In a study of 810 participants, one-third were taught how to lower their sodium intake and follow the DASH eating plan on their own. Most of them needed to lose weight as well. They followed the DASH eating plan at lower calorie levels and they increased their physical activity. Over the course of 18 months, participants lost weight and improved their blood pressure control.

JOSE HENRIQUEZ

" I was overweight. I was told by my doctor that if I kept it up I was going to develop high blood pressure and high blood cholesterol. The doctor sent me to a dietitian. She is the one who taught me the things that I had to do in order to eat right. It was hard at the beginning because once you have bad habits they are hard to break. Once I realized it was for my own good and no one was going to take care of me except me, I decided to start eating better. At home, we keep stuff like fruits, vegetables, and low-fat or fat-free milk in the house. My three daughters are beginning to learn how to eat right, and my little one loves vegetables like I do. "

If you're trying to lose weight, use the foods and serving guidelines in boxes 3 and 4 on pages 8 and 9. Aim for a caloric level that is lower than what you usually consume. In addition, you can make your diet lower in calories by using the tips in box 5. The best way to take off pounds is to do so gradually, get more physical activity, and eat a balanced diet that is lower in calories and fat. For some people at very high risk for heart disease or stroke, medication will be necessary. To develop a weight-loss or weight-maintenance program that works well for you, consult with your doctor or registered dietitian.

Combining the DASH eating plan with a regular physical activity program, such as walking or swimming, will help you both shed pounds and stay trim for the long term. You can do an activity for 30 minutes at one time, or choose shorter periods of at least 10 minutes each. (See box 6 on page 14.) The important thing is to total about 30 minutes of activity each day. (To avoid weight gain, try to total about 60 minutes per day.)

You should be aware that the DASH eating plan has more daily servings of fruits, vegetables, and whole grain foods than you may be used to eating. Because the plan is high in fiber, it can cause bloating and diarrhea in some persons. To avoid these problems, gradually increase your intake of fruit, vegetables, and whole grain foods.

This booklet gives menus and recipes from the DASH studies for both 2,300 and 1,500 milligrams of daily sodium intake. Twenty-three hundred milligrams of sodium equals about 6 grams, or 1 teaspoon, of table salt (sodium chloride); 1,500 milligrams of sodium equals about 4 grams, or $2/3$ teaspoon, of table salt.

The key to reducing salt intake is making wise food choices. Only a small amount of salt that we consume comes from the salt added at the table, and only small amounts of sodium occur naturally in food. Processed foods account for most of the salt and sodium Americans consume. So, be sure to read food labels to choose products lower in sodium. You may be surprised to find which foods have sodium. They include baked goods, certain cereals, soy sauce, seasoned salts, monosodium glutamate (MSG), baking soda, and some antacids—the range is wide.

How to Lower Calories on the DASH Eating Plan

The DASH eating plan can be adopted to promote weight loss. It is rich in lower-calorie foods, such as fruits and vegetables. You can make it lower in calories by replacing higher calorie foods such as sweets with more fruits and vegetables—and that also will make it easier for you to reach your DASH goals. Here are some examples:

To increase fruits—
- Eat a medium apple instead of four shortbread cookies. *You'll save 80 calories.*
- Eat 1/4 cup of dried apricots instead of a 2-ounce bag of pork rinds. *You'll save 230 calories.*

To increase vegetables—
- Have a hamburger that's 3 ounces of meat instead of 6 ounces. Add a 1/2-cup serving of carrots and a 1/2-cup serving of spinach. *You'll save more than 200 calories.*
- Instead of 5 ounces of chicken, have a stir fry with 2 ounces of chicken and 1 1/2 cups of raw vegetables. Use a small amount of vegetable oil. *You'll save 50 calories.*

To increase fat-free or low-fat milk products—
- Have a 1/2-cup serving of low-fat frozen yogurt instead of a 1/2-cup serving of full-fat ice cream. *You'll save about 70 calories.*

And don't forget these calorie-saving tips:
- Use fat-free or low-fat condiments.
- Use half as much vegetable oil, soft or liquid margarine, mayonnaise, or salad dressing, or choose available low-fat or fat-free versions.
- Eat smaller portions—cut back gradually.
- Choose fat-free or low-fat milk and milk products.
- Check the food labels to compare fat content in packaged foods— items marked fat-free or low-fat are not always lower in calories than their regular versions.
- Limit foods with lots of added sugar, such as pies, flavored yogurts, candy bars, ice cream, sherbet, regular soft drinks, and fruit drinks.
- Eat fruits canned in their own juice or in water.
- Add fruit to plain fat-free or low-fat yogurt.
- Snack on fruit, vegetable sticks, unbuttered and unsalted popcorn, or rice cakes.
- Drink water or club soda—zest it up with a wedge of lemon or lime.

BOX 6

Make a Dash for DASH

Thirty minutes of moderate-intensity physical activity each day can help.

- If your blood pressure is moderately elevated, 30 minutes of brisk walking on most days a week may be enough to keep you off medication.
- If you take medication for high blood pressure, 30 minutes of moderate physical activity can make your medication work more effectively and make you feel better.
- If you don't have high blood pressure, being physically active can help keep it that way. If you have normal blood pressure—but are not active—your chances of developing high blood pressure increase, especially as you get older or if you become overweight or obese or develop diabetes.

Getting started: Your physical activity program can be as simple as a 15-minute walk around the block each morning and evening. Gradually build up your program and set new goals to stay motivated. The important thing is to find something you enjoy, and do it safely. And remember—trying too hard at first can lead to injury and cause you to give up. If you have a chronic health problem or a family history of heart disease at an early age, be sure to talk with your doctor before launching a new physical activity program.

1. **Set a schedule and try to keep it.**
2. **Get a friend or family member to join you.** Motivate each other to keep it up.
3. **Cross-train.** Alternate between different activities so you don't strain one part of your body day after day.
4. **Set goals.**
5. **Reward yourself.** At the end of each month that you stay on your exercise program, reward yourself with something new—new clothes, a compact disc, a new book—something that will help keep you committed. But don't use food as a reward.

Because it is rich in fruits and vegetables, which are naturally lower in sodium than many other foods, the DASH eating plan makes it easier to consume less salt and sodium. Still, you may want to begin by adopting the DASH eating plan at the level of 2,300 milligrams of sodium per day and then further lower your sodium intake to 1,500 milligrams per day.

Boxes 7, 8, and 9 on pages 16–18 offer tips on how to reduce the salt and sodium content in your diet, and boxes 10 and 11 on pages 19 and 20 show how to use food labels to find lower sodium products.

The DASH eating plan also emphasizes potassium from food, especially fruits and vegetables, to help keep blood pressure levels healthy. A potassium-rich diet may help to reduce elevated or high blood pressure, but be sure to get your potassium from food sources, not from supplements. Many fruits and vegetables, some milk products, and fish are rich sources of potassium. (See box 12 on page 21.) However, fruits and vegetables are rich in the form of potassium (potassium with bicarbonate precursors) that favorably affects acid-base metabolism. This form of potassium may help to reduce risk of kidney stones and bone loss. While salt substitutes containing potassium are sometimes needed by persons on drug therapy for high blood pressure, these supplements can be harmful to people with certain medical conditions. Ask your doctor before trying salt substitutes or supplements.

Start the DASH eating plan today—it can help you prevent and control high blood pressure, has other health benefits for your heart, can be used to lose weight, and meets your nutritional needs.

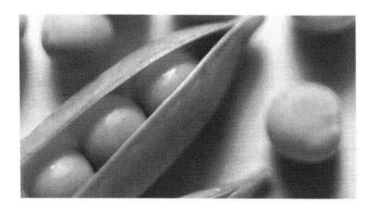

Where's the Sodium?

Only a small amount of sodium occurs naturally in foods. Most sodium is added during processing. The table below gives examples of sodium in some foods.

Food Groups	Sodium (mg)
Whole and other grains and grain products*	
Cooked cereal, rice, pasta, unsalted, 1/2 cup	0–5
Ready-to-eat cereal, 1 cup	0–360
Bread, 1 slice	110–175
Vegetables	
Fresh or frozen, cooked without salt, 1/2 cup	1–70
Canned or frozen with sauce, 1/2 cup	140–460
Tomato juice, canned, 1/2 cup	330
Fruit	
Fresh, frozen, canned, 1/2 cup	0–5
Low-fat or fat-free milk and milk products	
Milk, 1 cup	107
Yogurt, 1 cup	175
Natural cheeses, 1 1/2 oz	110–450
Process cheeses, 2 oz	600
Nuts, seeds, and legumes	
Peanuts, salted, 1/3 cup	120
Peanuts, unsalted, 1/3 cup	0–5
Beans, cooked from dried or frozen, without salt, 1/2 cup	0–5
Beans, canned, 1/2 cup	400
Lean meats, fish, and poultry	
Fresh meat, fish, poultry, 3 oz	30–90
Tuna canned, water pack, no salt added, 3 oz	35–45
Tuna canned, water pack, 3 oz	230–350
Ham, lean, roasted, 3 oz	1,020

* Whole grains are recommended for most grain servings.

BOX 8

Tips To Reduce Salt and Sodium

- Choose low- or reduced-sodium, or no-salt-added versions of foods and condiments when available.
- Choose fresh, frozen, or canned (low-sodium or no-salt-added) vegetables.
- Use fresh poultry, fish, and lean meat, rather than canned, smoked, or processed types.
- Choose ready-to-eat breakfast cereals that are lower in sodium.
- Limit cured foods (such as bacon and ham); foods packed in brine (such as pickles, pickled vegetables, olives, and sauerkraut); and condiments (such as mustard, horseradish, ketchup, and barbecue sauce). Limit even lower sodium versions of soy sauce and teriyaki sauce. Treat these condiments sparingly as you do table salt.
- Cook rice, pasta, and hot cereals without salt. Cut back on instant or flavored rice, pasta, and cereal mixes, which usually have added salt.
- Choose "convenience" foods that are lower in sodium. Cut back on frozen dinners, mixed dishes such as pizza, packaged mixes, canned soups or broths, and salad dressings—these often have a lot of sodium.
- Rinse canned foods, such as tuna and canned beans, to remove some of the sodium.
- Use spices instead of salt. In cooking and at the table, flavor foods with herbs, spices, lemon, lime, vinegar, or salt-free seasoning blends. Start by cutting salt in half.

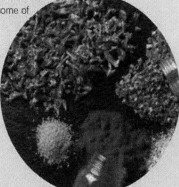

BOX 9

Reducing Salt and Sodium When Eating Out

- Ask how foods are prepared. Ask that they be prepared without added salt, MSG, or salt-containing ingredients. Most restaurants are willing to accommodate requests.
- Know the terms that indicate high sodium content: pickled, cured, smoked, soy sauce, broth.
- Move the salt shaker away.
- Limit condiments, such as mustard, ketchup, pickles, and sauces with salt-containing ingredients.
- Choose fruit or vegetables, instead of salty snack foods.

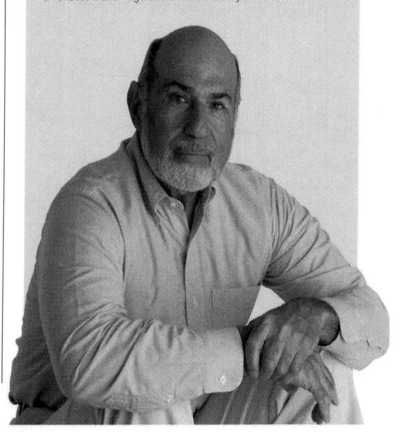

Compare Nutrition Facts Labels on Foods

Read the Nutrition Facts labels on foods to compare the amount of sodium in products. Look for the sodium content in milligrams and the Percent Daily Value. Aim for foods that are less than 5 percent of the Daily Value of sodium. Foods with 20 percent or more Daily Value of sodium are considered high. You can also check out the amounts of the other DASH goal nutrients.

Compare the food labels of these two versions of canned tomatoes. The regular canned tomatoes (right) have 15 times as much sodium as the low-sodium canned tomatoes.

Low-Sodium Canned Diced Tomatoes

Canned Diced Tomatoes

Nutrition Facts
Serving Size ¹/₂ cup (130g)
Servings Per Container 3¹/₂

Amount Per Serving

Calories 25	Calories from Fat 0

	% Daily Value*
Total Fat 0g	**0%**
Saturated Fat 0g	**0%**
Trans Fat 0g	
Cholesterol 0mg	**0%**
Sodium 10mg	**1%**
Potassium 270mg	**8%**
Total Carbohydrate 5g	**2%**
Dietary Fiber 1g	**4%**
Sugar 3g	
Protein 1g	

Vitamin A	5%	Vitamin C	30%
Calcium	4%	Iron	4%

*Percent Daily Values are based on a 2,000 calorie diet.

Nutrition Facts
Serving Size ¹/₂ cup (130g)
Servings Per Container 3¹/₂

Amount Per Serving

Calories 25	Calories from Fat 0

	% Daily Value*
Total Fat 0g	**0%**
Saturated Fat 0g	**0%**
Trans Fat 0g	
Cholesterol 0mg	**0%**
Sodium 150mg	**6%**
Potassium 230mg	**6%**
Total Carbohydrate 5g	**2%**
Dietary Fiber 1g	**4%**
Sugar 3g	
Protein 1g	

Vitamin A	5%	Vitamin C	20%
Calcium	4%	Iron	6%

*Percent Daily Values are based on a 2,000 calorie diet.

Label Language

Food labels can help you choose items lower in sodium, saturated fat, trans fat, cholesterol, and calories and higher in potassium and calcium. Look for the following label information on cans, boxes, bottles, bags, and other packaging:

Phrase	What It Means*
Sodium	
Sodium free or salt free	Less than 5 mg per serving
Very low sodium	35 mg or less of sodium per serving
Low sodium	140 mg or less of sodium per serving
Low-sodium meal	140 mg or less of sodium per 3½ oz (100 g)
Reduced or less sodium	At least 25 percent less sodium than the regular version
Light in sodium	50 percent less sodium than the regular version
Unsalted or no salt added	No salt added to the product during processing (this is not a sodium-free food)
Fat	
Fat-free	Less than 0.5 g per serving
Low saturated fat	1 g or less per serving and 15% or less of calories from saturated fat
Low-fat	3 g or less per serving
Reduced fat	At least 25 percent less fat than the regular version
Light in fat	Half the fat compared to the regular version

* Small serving sizes (50 g) or meals and main dishes are based on various weights in grams versus a serving size.

Where's the Potassium?

Potassium comes from a variety of food sources. The table below gives examples of potassium in some foods.

Food Groups	Potassium (mg)
Vegetables	
Potato, 1 medium	926
Sweet Potato, 1 medium	540
Spinach, cooked, 1/2 cup	290
Zucchini, cooked, 1/2 cup	280
Tomato, fresh, 1/2 cup	210
Kale, cooked, 1/2 cup	150
Romaine lettuce, 1 cup	140
Mushrooms, 1/2 cup	110
Cucumber, 1/2 cup	80
Fruit	
Banana, 1 medium	420
Apricots, 1/4 cup	380
Orange, 1 medium	237
Cantaloupe chunks, 1/2 cup	214
Apple, 1 medium	150
Nuts, seeds, and legumes	
Cooked soybeans, 1/2 cup	440
Cooked lentils, 1/2 cup	370
Cooked kidney beans, 1/2 cup	360
Cooked split peas, 1/2 cup	360
Almonds, roasted, 1/3 cup	310
Walnuts, roasted, 1/3 cup	190
Sunflower seeds, roasted, 2 Tbsp	124
Peanuts, roasted, 1/3 cup	120
Low-fat or fat-free milk and milk products	
Milk, 1 cup	380
Yogurt, 1 cup	370
Lean meats, fish, and poultry	
Fish (cod, halibut, rockfish, trout, tuna), 3 oz	200–400
Pork tenderloin, 3 oz	370
Beef tenderloin, chicken, turkey, 3 oz	210

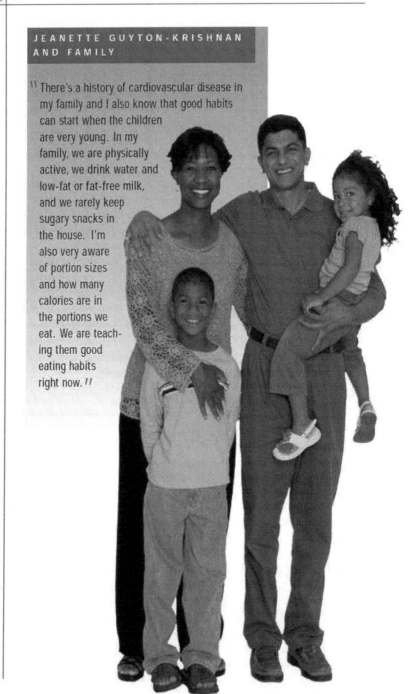

JEANETTE GUYTON-KRISHNAN AND FAMILY

" There's a history of cardiovascular disease in my family and I also know that good habits can start when the children are very young. In my family, we are physically active, we drink water and low-fat or fat-free milk, and we rarely keep sugary snacks in the house. I'm also very aware of portion sizes and how many calories are in the portions we eat. We are teaching them good eating habits right now. "

How Can I Get Started on the DASH Eating Plan?

It's easy. Reading the "Getting Started" suggestions in box 13 should help you along the way. The DASH eating plan requires no special foods and has no hard-to-follow recipes. One way to begin is by seeing how DASH compares with your current food habits. Use the "What's On Your Plate?" form. (See box 14 on page 26.) Fill it in for 1–2 days and see how it compares with the DASH plan. This will help you see what changes you need to make in your food choices.

Remember that on some days the foods you eat may add up to more than the recommended servings from one food group and less from another. Similarly, you may have too much sodium on a particular day. But don't worry. Try your best to keep the average of several days close to the DASH eating plan and the sodium level recommended for you.

Use the menus that begin on page 30 if you want to follow the menus similar to those used in the DASH trial—or make up your own using your favorite foods. In fact, your entire family can eat meals using the DASH eating plan. Use box 3 on page 8 to choose your favorite foods from each food group based on your calorie needs as described in the 2005 "U.S. Dietary Guidelines for Americans."

The Dietary Guidelines determined that the DASH eating plan is an example of a healthy eating plan and recommends it as a plan that not only meets your nutritional needs but can accommodate varied types of cuisines and special needs.

Remember that the DASH eating plan used along with other lifestyle changes can help you prevent and control your blood pressure. Important lifestyle recommendations for you include: achieve and maintain a healthy weight, participate in your favorite regular physical activity, and, if you drink, use moderation in alcohol consumption (defined as up to one drink per day for women and up to two drinks per day for men).

One important note: If you take medication to control high blood pressure, you should not stop using it. Follow the DASH eating plan and talk with your doctor about your medication treatment. The tips in box 15 on page 27 can help you continue to follow the DASH eating plan and make other healthy lifestyle changes for a lifetime.

Getting Started

It's easy to adopt the DASH eating plan. Here are some ways to get started:

Change gradually

- If you now eat one or two vegetables a day, add a serving at lunch and another at dinner.
- If you don't eat fruit now or have juice only at breakfast, add a serving to your meals or have it as a snack.
- Gradually increase your use of fat-free and low-fat milk and milk products to three servings a day. For example, drink milk with lunch or dinner, instead of soda, sugar-sweetened tea, or alcohol. Choose fat-free (skim) or low-fat (1 percent) milk and milk products to reduce your intake of saturated fat, total fat, cholesterol, and calories and to increase your calcium.
- Read the Nutrition Facts label on margarines and salad dressings to choose those lowest in saturated fat and trans fat.

Treat meats as one part of the whole meal, instead of the focus

- Limit lean meats to 6 ounces a day—all that's needed. Have only 3 ounces at a meal, which is about the size of a deck of cards.
- If you now eat large portions of meats, cut them back gradually— by a half or a third at each meal.
- Include two or more vegetarian-style (meatless) meals each week.
- Increase servings of vegetables, brown rice, whole wheat pasta, and cooked dry beans in meals. Try casseroles, whole wheat pasta, and stir-fry dishes, which have less meat and more vegetables, grains, and dry beans.

Use fruits or other foods low in saturated fat, trans fat, cholesterol, sodium, sugar, and calories as desserts and snacks

- Fruits and other lower fat foods offer great taste and variety. Use fruits canned in their own juice or packed in water. Fresh fruits require little or no preparation. Dried fruits are a good choice to carry with you or to have ready in the car.
- Try these snacks ideas: unsalted rice cakes; nuts mixed with raisins; graham crackers; fat-free and low-fat yogurt and frozen yogurt; popcorn with no salt or butter added; raw vegetables.

Try these other tips

- Choose whole grain foods for most grain servings to get added nutrients, such as minerals and fiber. For example, choose whole wheat bread or whole grain cereals.
- If you have trouble digesting milk and milk products, try taking lactase enzyme pills (available at drugstores and groceries) with the milk products. Or, buy lactose-free milk, which has the lactase enzyme already added to it.
- If you are allergic to nuts, use seeds or legumes (cooked dried beans or peas).
- Use fresh, frozen, or low-sodium canned vegetables and fruits.

Use the form in box 14 to track your food and physical activities habits before you start on the DASH eating plan or to see how you're doing after a few weeks. To record more than 1 day, just copy the form. Total each day's food groups and compare what you ate with the DASH eating plan. To see how the form looks completed, check the menus that start on page 30.

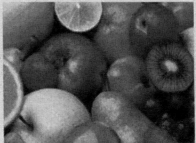

BOX 14

What's on Your Plate?
How Much Are You Moving?

Date:			Number of Servings by DASH Food Group								
Food	Amount (serving size)	Sodium (mg)	Grains	Vegetables	Fruits	Milk Products	Meats, fish, and poultry	Nuts, seeds, and legumes	Fats and oils	Sweets and added sugars
Example: whole wheat bread, with soft (tub) margarine	2 slices 2 tsp	299 52	2						2	
Breakfast										
Lunch										
Dinner										
Snacks										
Day's Totals										
Compare yours with the DASH eating plan at 2,000 calories.		2,300 or 1,500 mg per day	6–8 per day	4–5 per day	4–5 per day	2–3 per day	6 or less per day	4–5 per week	2–3 per day	5 or less per week
Physical Activity Log Record your minutes per day for each activity. Aim for at least 30 minutes of moderate-intensity physical activity on most days of the week.										

BOX 15

Making the DASH to Good Health

The DASH plan is a new way of eating—for a lifetime. If you slip from the eating plan for a few days, don't let it keep you from reaching your health goals. Get back on track. Here's how:

Ask yourself why you got off-track.
Was it at a party? Were you feeling stress at home or work? Find out what triggered your sidetrack and start again with the DASH plan.

Don't worry about a slip.
Everyone slips—especially when learning something new. Remember that changing your lifestyle is a long-term process.

See if you tried to do too much at once.
Often, those starting a new lifestyle try to change too much at once. Instead, change one or two things at a time. Slowly but surely is the best way to succeed.

Break the process down into small steps.
This not only keeps you from trying to do too much at once, but also keeps the changes simpler. Break complex goals into smaller, simpler steps, each of which is attainable.

Write it down.
Use the table in box 14 to keep track of what you eat and what you're doing. This can help you find the problem. Keep track for several days. You may find, for instance, that you eat high-fat foods while watching television. If so, you could start keeping a substitute snack on hand to eat instead of the high-fat foods. This record also helps you be sure you're getting enough of each food group and physical activity each day.

Celebrate success.
Treat yourself to a nonfood treat for your accomplishments.

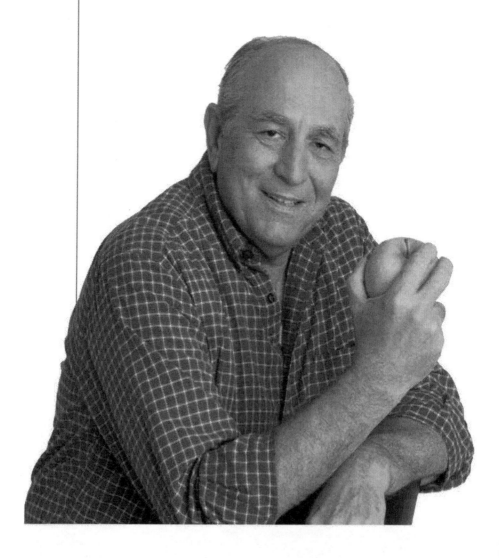

A Week With
the DASH Eating Plan

Here is a week of menus from the DASH eating plan. The menus allow you to have a daily sodium level of either 2,300 mg or, by making the noted changes, 1,500 mg. You'll also find that the menus sometimes call for you to use lower sodium, low-fat, fat-free, or reduced fat versions of products.

The menus are based on 2,000 calories a day—serving sizes should be increased or decreased for other calorie levels. To ease the calculations, some of the serving sizes have been rounded off. Also, some items may be in too small a quantity to have a listed food group serving. Recipes for starred items are given on the later pages. Some of these recipes give changes that can be used to lower their sodium level. Use the changes if you want to follow the DASH eating plan at 1,500 milligrams of sodium per day.

Abbreviations:
oz = ounce
tsp = teaspoon
Tbsp = tablespoon
g = gram
mg = milligram

Day 1

2,300 mg Sodium Menu	Sodium (mg)	Substitution To Reduce Sodium to 1,500 mg	Sodium (mg)
Breakfast			
³/4 cup bran flakes cereal:	220	³/4 cup shredded wheat cereal	1
1 medium banana	1		
1 cup low-fat milk	107		
1 slice whole wheat bread:	149		
1 tsp soft (tub) margarine	26	1 tsp unsalted soft (tub) margarine	0
1 cup orange juice	5		
Lunch			
³/4 cup chicken salad:*	179	Remove salt from the recipe*	120
2 slices whole wheat bread	299		
1 Tbsp Dijon mustard	373	1 Tbsp regular mustard	175
salad:			
¹/2 cup fresh cucumber slices	1		
¹/2 cup tomato wedges	5		
1 Tbsp sunflower seeds	0		
1 tsp Italian dressing, low calorie	43		
¹/2 cup fruit cocktail, juice pack	5		
Dinner			
3 oz beef, eye of the round:	35		
2 Tbsp beef gravy, fat-free	165		
1 cup green beans, sautéed with:	12		
¹/2 tsp canola oil	0		
1 small baked potato:	14		
1 Tbsp sour cream, fat-free	21		
1 Tbsp grated natural cheddar cheese, reduced fat	67	1 Tbsp natural cheddar cheese, reduced fat, low sodium	1
1 Tbsp chopped scallions	1		
1 small whole wheat roll:	148		
1 tsp soft (tub) margarine	26	1 tsp unsalted soft (tub) margarine	0
1 small apple	1		
1 cup low-fat milk	107		
Snacks			
¹/3 cup almonds, unsalted	0		
¹/4 cup raisins	4		
¹/2 cup fruit yogurt, fat-free, no sugar added	86		
Totals	**2,101**		**1,507**

* Recipe on page 45

Nutrients Per Day	Sodium Level	
	2,300 mg	1,500 mg
Calories	2,062	2,037
Total fat	63 g	59 g
Calories from fat	28 %	26 %
Saturated fat	13 g	12 g
Calories from saturated fat	6 %	5 %
Cholesterol	155 mg	155 mg
Sodium	2,101 mg	1,507 mg

Number of Servings by DASH Food Group

Grains	Vegetables	Fruits	Milk Products	Meats, Fish, and Poultry	Nuts, Seeds, and Legumes	Fats and Oils	Sweets and Added Sugars
1							
		1					
			1				
1							
		2				1	
				3		1	
2							
	1						
	1						
					1/2		
		1					
				3			
	2						
	1					1/2	
1							
		1				1	
			1				
					1		
		1					
			1/2				
5	5	6	2½	6	1½	3½	0

Nutrients Per Day	Sodium Level	
	2,300 mg	1,500 mg
Carbohydrate	284 g	284 g
Protein	114 g	115 g
Calcium	1,220 mg	1,218 mg
Magnesium	594 mg	580 mg
Potassium	4,909 mg	4,855 mg
Fiber	37 g	36 g

Day 2

2,300 mg Sodium Menu	Sodium (mg)	Substitution To Reduce Sodium to 1,500 mg	Sodium (mg)
Breakfast			
¹/₂ cup instant oatmeal	54	¹/₂ cup regular oatmeal with 1 tsp cinnamon	5
1 mini whole wheat bagel:	84		
1 Tbsp peanut butter	81		
1 medium banana	1		
1 cup low-fat milk	107		
Lunch			
chicken breast sandwich:			
3 oz chicken breast, skinless	65		
2 slices whole wheat bread	299		
1 slice (³/₄ oz) natural cheddar cheese, reduced fat	202	1 slice (³/₄ oz) natural Swiss cheese, low sodium	3
1 large leaf romaine lettuce	1		
2 slices tomato	2		
1 Tbsp mayonnaise, low-fat	101		
1 cup cantaloupe chunks	26		
1 cup apple juice	21		
Dinner			
1 cup spaghetti:	1		
³/₄ cup vegetarian spaghetti sauce*	479	Substitute low-sodium tomato paste (6 oz) in recipe*	253
3 Tbsp Parmesan cheese	287		
spinach salad:			
1 cup fresh spinach leaves	24		
¹/₄ cup fresh carrots, grated	19		
¹/₄ cup fresh mushrooms, sliced	1		
1 Tbsp vinaigrette dressing†	1		
¹/₂ cup corn, cooked from frozen	1		
¹/₂ cup canned pears, juice pack	5		
Snacks			
¹/₃ cup almonds, unsalted	0		
¹/₄ cup dried apricots	3		
1 cup fruit yogurt, fat-free, no sugar added	173		
Totals	**2,035**		**1,560**

* Recipe on page 46
† Recipe on page 47

Nutrients Per Day	Sodium Level	
	2,300 mg	1,500 mg
Calories	2,027	2,078
Total fat	64 g	68 g
Calories from fat	28 %	30 %
Saturated fat	13 g	16 g
Calories from saturated fat	6 %	7 %
Cholesterol	114 mg	129 mg
Sodium	2,035 mg	1,560 mg

	Number of Servings by DASH Food Group						
Grains	Vegetables	Fruits	Milk Products	Meats, Fish, and Poultry	Nuts, Seeds, and Legumes	Fats and Oils	Sweets and Added Sugars
1							
1					1/2		
		1					
				1			
				3			
2			1/2				
	1/4						
	1/2					1	
		2					
		2					
2							
	1 1/2						
			1/2				
	1						
	1/2						
	1/2					1/2	
	1						
		1					
					1		
		1					
			1				
6	5 1/4	7	3	3	1 1/2	1 1/2	0

	Sodium Level	
Nutrients Per Day	2,300 mg	1,500 mg
Carbohydrate	288 g	290 g
Protein	99 g	100 g
Calcium	1,370 mg	1,334 mg
Magnesium	535 mg	542 mg
Potassium	4,715 mg	4,721 mg
Fiber	34 g	34 g

Day 3

2,300 mg Sodium Menu	Sodium (mg)	Substitution To Reduce Sodium to 1,500 mg	Sodium (mg)
Breakfast			
3/4 cup bran flakes cereal:	220	2 cups puffed wheat cereal	1
1 medium banana	1		
1 cup low-fat milk	107		
1 slice whole wheat bread:	149		
1 tsp soft (tub) margarine	26	1 tsp unsalted soft (tub) margarine	0
1 cup orange juice	6		
Lunch			
beef barbeque sandwich:			
2 oz beef, eye of round	26		
1 Tbsp barbeque sauce	156		
2 slices (1 1/2 oz) natural cheddar cheese, reduced fat	405	1 1/2 oz natural cheddar cheese, reduced fat, low sodium	9
1 hamburger bun	183		
1 large leaf romaine lettuce	1		
2 slices tomato	2		
1 cup new potato salad*	17		
1 medium orange	0		
Dinner			
3 oz cod:	70		
1 tsp lemon juice	1		
1/2 cup brown rice	5		
1 cup spinach, cooked from frozen, sautéed with:	184		
1 tsp canola oil	0		
1 Tbsp almonds, slivered	0		
1 small cornbread muffin, made with oil:	119		
1 tsp soft (tub) margarine	26	1 tsp unsalted soft (tub) margarine	0
Snacks			
1 cup fruit yogurt, fat-free, no added sugar:	173		
1 Tbsp sunflower seeds, unsalted	0		
2 large graham cracker rectangles:	156		
1 Tbsp peanut butter	81		
Totals	**2,114**		**1,447**

* Recipe on page 48

Nutrients Per Day	Sodium Level	
	2,300 mg	1,500 mg
Calories	1,997	1,995
Total fat	56 g	52 g
Calories from fat	25 %	24 %
Saturated fat	12 g	11 g
Calories from saturated fat	6 %	5 %
Cholesterol	140 mg	140 mg
Sodium	2,114 mg	1,447 mg

				Number of Servings by DASH Food Group			
Grains	Vegetables	Fruits	Milk Products	Meats, Fish, and Poultry	Nuts, Seeds, and Legumes	Fats and Oils	Sweets and Added Sugars
1		1					
				1			
1							
						1	
		2					
				2			
			1				
2							
	1/4						
	1/2						
	2						
		1					
				3			
1							
	2						
						1	
1					1/4		
						1	
			1				
					1/2		
1							
					1/2		
7	4 3/4	4	3	5	1 1/4	3	0

Nutrients Per Day	Sodium Level	
	2,300 mg	1,500 mg
Carbohydrate	289 g	283 g
Protein	103 g	104 g
Calcium	1,537 mg	1,524 mg
Magnesium	630 mg	598 mg
Potassium	4,676 mg	4,580 mg
Fiber	34 g	31 g

Day 4

2,300 mg Sodium Menu	Sodium (mg)	Substitution To Reduce Sodium to 1,500 mg	Sodium (mg)
Breakfast			
1 slice whole wheat bread:	149		
1 tsp soft (tub) margarine	26	1 tsp unsalted soft (tub) margarine	0
1 cup fruit yogurt, fat-free, no added sugar	173		
1 medium peach	0		
1/2 cup grape juice	4		
Lunch			
ham and cheese sandwich:			
2 oz ham, low-fat, low sodium	549	2 oz roast beef tenderloin	23
1 slice (3/4 oz) natural cheddar cheese, reduced fat	202	1 slice (3/4 oz) natural cheddar cheese, reduced fat, low sodium	4
2 slices whole wheat bread	299		
1 large leaf romaine lettuce	1		
2 slices tomato	2		
1 Tbsp mayonnaise, low-fat	101		
1 cup carrot sticks	84		
Dinner			
chicken and Spanish rice*	341	substitute low-sodium tomato sauce (4 oz) in recipe*	215
1 cup green peas, sautéed with:	115		
1 tsp canola oil	0		
1 cup cantaloupe chunks	26		
1 cup low-fat milk	107		
Snacks			
1/3 cup almonds, unsalted	0		
1 cup apple juice	21		
1/4 cup apricots	3		
1 cup low-fat milk	107		
Totals	**2,312**		**1,436**

* *Recipe on page 49*

Nutrients Per Day	Sodium Level	
	2,300 mg	1,500 mg
Calories	2,024	2,045
Total fat	59 g	59 g
Calories from fat	26 %	26 %
Saturated fat	12 g	12 g
Calories from saturated fat	5 %	5 %
Cholesterol	148 mg	150 mg
Sodium	2,312 mg	1,436 mg

Number of Servings by DASH Food Group

Grains	Vegetables	Fruits	Milk Products	Meats, Fish, and Poultry	Nuts, Seeds, and Legumes	Fats and Oils	Sweets and Added Sugars
1						1	
			1				
		1					
		1					
				2			
			1/2				
2							
	1/4						
	1/2						
	2					1	
1				3			
	2						
		2				1	
			1				
					1		
		2					
		1					
			1				
4	**4³/4**	**7**	**3¹/2**	**5**	**1**	**3**	**0**

	Sodium Level	
Nutrients Per Day	**2,300 mg**	**1,500 mg**
Carbohydrate	279 g	278 g
Protein	110 g	116 g
Calcium	1,417 mg	1,415 mg
Magnesium	538 mg	541 mg
Potassium	4,575 mg	4,559 mg
Fiber	35 g	35 g

Day 5

2,300 mg Sodium Menu	Sodium (mg)	Substitution To Reduce Sodium to 1,500 mg	Sodium (mg)
Breakfast			
1 cup whole grain oat rings cereal:	273	1 cup frosted shredded wheat	4
1 medium banana	1		
1 cup low-fat milk	107		
1 medium raisin bagel:	272		
1 Tbsp peanut butter	81	1 Tbsp peanut butter, unsalted	3
1 cup orange juice	5		
Lunch			
tuna salad plate:			
1/2 cup tuna salad*	171		
1 large leaf romaine lettuce	1		
1 slice whole wheat bread	149	6 whole wheat crackers, low sodium	53
cucumber salad:			
1 cup fresh cucumber slices	2		
1/2 cup tomato wedges	5		
1 Tbsp vinaigrette dressing	133	2 Tbsp yogurt dressing, fat-free†	66
1/2 cup cottage cheese, low-fat:	459		
1/2 cup canned pineapple, juice pack	1		
1 Tbsp almonds, unsalted	0		
Dinner			
3 oz turkey meatloaf‡	205	substitute low-sodium ketchup in recipe‡	74
1 small baked potato:	14		
1 Tbsp sour cream, fat-free	21		
1 Tbsp natural cheddar cheese, reduced fat, grated	67	1 Tbsp natural cheddar cheese, reduced fat, and low sodium	1
1 scallion stalk, chopped	1		
1 cup collard greens, sautéed with:	85		
1 tsp canola oil	0		
1 small whole wheat roll	148	6 small melba toast crackers, unsalted	1
1 medium peach	0		
Snacks			
1 cup fruit yogurt, fat-free, no added sugar	173		
2 Tbsp sunflower seeds, unsalted	0		
Totals	**2,373**		**1,519**

* Recipe on page 50
† Recipe on page 51
‡ Recipe on page 50

Nutrients Per Day	Sodium Level	
	2,300 mg	1,500 mg
Calories	1,976	2,100
Total fat	57 g	52 g
Calories from fat	26 %	22 %
Saturated fat	11 g	11 g
Calories from saturated fat	5 %	5 %
Cholesterol	158 mg	158 mg
Sodium	2,373 mg	1,519 mg

Grains	Vegetables	Fruits	Milk Products	Meats, Fish, and Poultry	Nuts, Seeds, and Legumes	Fats and Oils	Sweets and Added Sugars
1							
		1					
			1				
2							
					1/2		
		2					
				3			
	1/4						
1							
	2						
	1						
						1	
		1	1/4				
					1/4		
				3			
	1						
	2						
1						1	
		1					
			1				
					1		
5	6 1/4	5	2 1/4	6	1 3/4	2	0

Nutrients Per Day	Sodium Level	
	2,300 mg	1,500 mg
Carbohydrate	275 g	314 g
Protein	111 g	114 g
Calcium	1,470 mg	1,412 mg
Magnesium	495 mg	491 mg
Potassium	4,769 mg	4,903 mg
Fiber	30 g	31 g

Day 6

2,300 mg Sodium Menu	Sodium (mg)	Substitution To Reduce Sodium to 1,500 mg	Sodium (mg)	
Breakfast				
1 low-fat granola bar	81			
1 medium banana	1			
1/2 cup fruit yogurt, fat-free, no sugar added	86			
1 cup orange juice	5			
1 cup low-fat milk	107			
Lunch				
turkey breast sandwich:				
3 oz turkey breast	48			
2 slices whole wheat bread	299			
1 large leaf romaine lettuce	1			
2 slices tomato	2			
2 tsp mayonnaise, low-fat	67			
1 Tbsp Dijon mustard	373	1 Tbsp regular mustard	175	
1 cup steamed broccoli, cooked from frozen	11			
1 medium orange	0			
Dinner				
3 oz spicy baked fish*	50			
1 cup scallion rice†	18			
spinach sauté:				
1/2 cup spinach, cooked from frozen, sautéed with:	92			
2 tsp canola oil	0			
1 Tbsp almonds, slivered, unsalted	0			
1 cup carrots, cooked from frozen	84			
1 small whole wheat roll:	148			
1 tsp soft (tub) margarine	26			
1 small cookie	60			
Snacks				
2 Tbsp peanuts, unsalted	1			
1 cup low-fat milk	107			
1/4 cup dried apricots	3			
Totals	**1,671**		**1,472**	

* Recipe on page 52
† Recipe on page 53

Nutrients Per Day	Sodium Level	
	2,300 mg	1,500 mg
Calories	1,939	1,935
Total fat	58 g	57 g
Calories from fat	27 %	27 %
Saturated fat	12 g	12 g
Calories from saturated fat	6 %	6 %
Cholesterol	171 mg	171 mg
Sodium	1,671 mg	1,472 mg

Number of Servings by DASH Food Group

Grains	Vegetables	Fruits	Milk Products	Meats, Fish, and Poultry	Nuts, Seeds, and Legumes	Fats and Oils	Sweets and Added Sugars
1							
		1					
			1/2				
		2					
			1				
				3			
2	1/4						
	1/2						
						2/3	
	2						
		1					
				3			
2							
	1						
						2	
					1/4		
	2						
1							
						1	
							1
					1/2		
			1				
		1					
6	5 3/4	5	2 1/2	6	3/4	3 2/3	1

Nutrients Per Day	Sodium Level	
	2,300 mg	1,500 mg
Carbohydrate	268 g	268 g
Protein	105 g	105 g
Calcium	1,210 mg	1,214 mg
Magnesium	548 mg	545 mg
Potassium	4,710 mg	4,710 mg
Fiber	36 g	36 g

Day 7

2,300 mg Sodium Menu	Sodium (mg)	Substitution To Reduce Sodium to 1,500 mg	Sodium (mg)	
Breakfast				
1 cup whole grain oat rings:	273	1 cup regular oatmeal	5	
1 medium banana	1			
1 cup low-fat milk	107			
1 cup fruit yogurt, fat-free, no sugar added	173			
Lunch				
tuna salad sandwich:				
½ cup tuna, drained, rinsed	39			
1 Tbsp mayonnaise, low-fat	101			
1 large leaf romaine lettuce	1			
2 slices tomato	2			
2 slices whole wheat bread	299			
1 medium apple	1			
1 cup low-fat milk	107			
Dinner				
⅙ recipe zucchini lasagna:*	368	substitute cottage cheese, low-fat, no salt added in recipe*	165	
salad:				
1 cup fresh spinach leaves	24			
1 cup tomato wedges	9			
2 Tbsp croutons, seasoned	62			
1 Tbsp vinaigrette dressing, reduced calorie	133	1 Tbsp low-sodium vinaigrette dressing, from recipe†	1	
1 Tbsp sunflower seeds	0			
1 small whole wheat roll:	148			
1 tsp soft (tub) margarine	45	1 tsp unsalted soft (tub) margarine	0	
1 cup grape juice	8			
Snacks				
⅓ cup almonds, unsalted	0			
¼ cup dry apricots	3			
6 whole wheat crackers	166			
Totals	**2,069**		**1,421**	

* *Recipe on page 54*
† *Recipe on page 47*

Nutrients Per Day	Sodium Level	
	2,300 mg	1,500 mg
Calories	1,993	1,988
Total fat	64 g	60 g
Calories from fat	29 %	27 %
Saturated fat	13 g	13 g
Calories from saturated fat	6 %	6 %
Cholesterol	71 mg	72 mg
Sodium	2,069 mg	1,421 mg

				Number of Servings by DASH Food Group			
Grains	Vegetables	Fruits	Milk Products	Meats, Fish, and Poultry	Nuts, Seeds, and Legumes	Fats and Oils	Sweets and Added Sugars
1		1					
			1				
			1				
				3			
	1/4					1	
2	1/2						
		1					
			1				
3	1		1				
	1						
1/4	2						
						1/2	
1					1/2		
		2				1	
					1		
		1					
1							
8 1/4	4 3/4	5	4	3	1 1/2	2 1/2	0

	Sodium Level	
Nutrients Per Day	**2,300 mg**	**1,500 mg**
Carbohydrate	283 g	285 g
Protein	93 g	97 g
Calcium	1,616 mg	1,447 mg
Magnesium	537 mg	553 mg
Potassium	4,693 mg	4,695 mg
Fiber	32 g	33 g

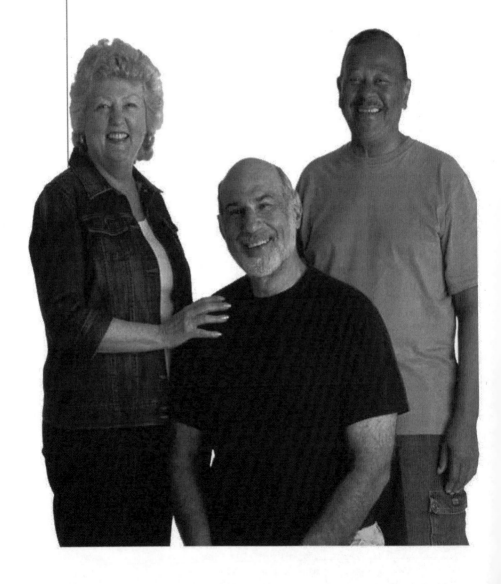

Recipes for Heart Health

Here are some recipes to help you cook up a week of tasty, heart healthy meals. If you're following the DASH eating plan at 1,500 milligrams of sodium per day or just want to reduce your sodium intake, use the suggested recipe changes.

Day 1

Chicken Salad

3¼	cups	chicken breast, cooked, cubed, and skinless
¼	cup	celery, chopped
1	Tbsp	lemon juice
½	tsp	onion powder
⅛	tsp	salt*
3	Tbsp	mayonnaise, low-fat

1. Bake chicken, cut into cubes, and refrigerate.
2. In a large bowl combine rest of ingredients, add chilled chicken and mix well.

Makes 5 servings
Serving Size: ¾ cup
Per Serving:

Calories	176	Carbohydrate	2 g
Total Fat	6 g	Calcium	16 mg
Saturated Fat	2 g	Magnesium	25 mg
Cholesterol	77 mg	Potassium	236 mg
Sodium	179 mg	Fiber	0 g
Protein	27 g		

* To reduce sodium, omit the ⅛ tsp of added salt.
  New sodium content for each serving is 120 mg.

Day 2

Vegetarian Spaghetti Sauce

2	Tbsp	olive oil
2	small	onions, chopped
3	cloves	garlic, chopped
1¼	cups	zucchini, sliced
1	Tbsp	oregano, dried
1	Tbsp	basil, dried
1	8 oz can	tomato sauce
1	6 oz can	tomato paste*
2	medium	tomatoes, chopped
1	cup	water

1. In a medium skillet, heat oil. Sauté onions, garlic, and zucchini in oil for 5 minutes on medium heat.
2. Add remaining ingredients and simmer covered for 45 minutes. Serve over spaghetti.

Makes 6 servings
Serving Size: ¾ cup
Per Serving:

Calories	105	Carbohydrate	15 g
Total Fat	5 g	Calcium	49 mg
Saturated Fat	1 g	Magnesium	35 mg
Cholesterol	0 mg	Potassium	686 mg
Sodium	479 mg	Fiber	4 g
Protein	3 g		

* To reduce sodium, use a 6-oz can of low-sodium tomato paste. New sodium content for each serving is 253 mg.

Vinaigrette Salad Dressing

1	bulb	garlic, separated and peeled
1/2	cup	water
1	Tbsp	red wine vinegar
1/4	tsp	honey
1	Tbsp	virgin olive oil
1/4	tsp	black pepper

1. Place the garlic cloves into a small saucepan and pour enough water (about 1/2 cup) to cover them.
2. Bring water to a boil, then reduce heat and simmer until garlic is tender, about 15 minutes.
3. Reduce the liquid to 2 Tbsp and increase the heat for 3 minutes.
4. Pour the contents into a small sieve over a bowl, and with a wooden spoon, mash the garlic through the sieve into the bowl.
5. Whisk the vinegar into the garlic mixture; incorporate the oil and seasoning.

Makes 4 servings
Serving Size: 2 Tbsp
Per Serving:

Calories	33	Carbohydrate	1 g
Total Fat	3 g	Calcium	3 mg
Saturated Fat	1 g	Magnesium	1 mg
Cholesterol	0 mg	Potassium	6 mg
Sodium	1 mg	Fiber	0 g
Protein	0 g		

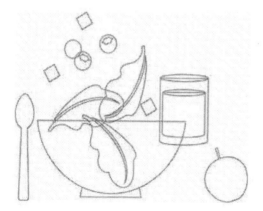

Day 3

New Potato Salad

16	small	new potatoes (5 cups)
2	Tbsp	olive oil
1/4	cup	green onions, chopped
1/4	tsp	black pepper
1	tsp	dill weed, dried

1. Thoroughly clean potatoes with vegetable brush and water.
2. Boil potatoes for 20 minutes or until tender.
3. Drain and cool potatoes for 20 minutes.
4. Cut potatoes into quarters and mix with olive oil, onions, and spices.
5. Refrigerate until ready to serve.

Makes 5 servings
Serving Size: 1 cup
Per Serving:

Calories	196	Carbohydrate	34 g
Total Fat	6 g	Calcium	31 mg
Saturated Fat	1 g	Magnesium	46 mg
Cholesterol	0 mg	Potassium	861 mg
Sodium	17 mg	Fiber	4 g
Protein	4 g		

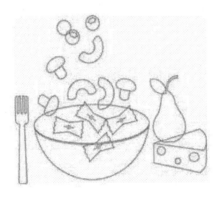

Chicken and Spanish Rice

1	cup	onions, chopped
3/4	cup	green peppers
2	tsp	vegetable oil
1	8 oz can	tomato sauce*
1	tsp	parsley, chopped
1/2	tsp	black pepper
1 1/4	tsp	garlic, minced
5	cups	cooked brown rice (cooked in unsalted water)
3 1/2	cups	chicken breasts, cooked, skin and bone removed, and diced

1. In a large skillet, sauté onions and green peppers in oil for 5 minutes on medium heat.
2. Add tomato sauce and spices. Heat through.
3. Add cooked rice and chicken. Heat through.

Makes 5 servings
Serving Size: 1 1/2 cup
Per Serving:

Calories	428	Carbohydrate	52 g
Total Fat	8 g	Calcium	50 mg
Saturated Fat	2 g	Magnesium	122 mg
Cholesterol	80 mg	Potassium	545 mg
Sodium	341 mg	Fiber	8 g
Protein	35 g		

* To reduce sodium, use one 4-oz can of low-sodium tomato sauce and one 4-oz can of regular tomato sauce. New sodium content for each serving is 215 mg.

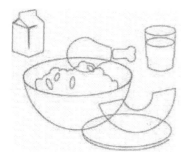

Day 5

Tuna Salad

2	6 oz cans	tuna, water pack
1/2	cup	raw celery, chopped
1/3	cup	green onions, chopped
6 1/2	Tbsp	mayonnaise, low-fat

1. Rinse and drain tuna for 5 minutes. Break apart with a fork.
2. Add celery, onion, and mayonnaise and mix well.

Makes 5 servings
Serving Size: 1/2 cup
Per Serving:

Calories	138	Carbohydrate	2 g
Total Fat	7 g	Calcium	17 mg
Saturated Fat	1 g	Magnesium	19 mg
Cholesterol	25 mg	Potassium	198 mg
Sodium	171 mg	Fiber	0 g
Protein	16 g		

Day 5

Turkey Meatloaf

1	pound	lean ground turkey
1/2	cup	regular oats, dry
1	large	egg, whole
1	Tbsp	onion, dehydrated flakes
1/4	cup	ketchup*

1. Combine all ingredients and mix well.
2. Bake in a loaf pan at 350 °F for 25 minutes or to an internal temperature of 165 °F.
3. Cut into five slices and serve.

Makes 5 servings
Serving Size: 1 slice (3 oz)
Per Serving:

Calories	191	Carbohydrate	9 g
Total Fat	7 g	Calcium	24 mg
Saturated Fat	2 g	Magnesium	33 mg
Cholesterol	103 mg	Potassium	268 mg
Sodium	205 mg	Fiber	1 g
Protein	23 g		

* To reduce sodium, use low-sodium ketchup.
New sodium content for each serving is 74 mg.

Day 5

Yogurt Salad Dressing

8	oz	plain yogurt, fat-free
1/4	cup	mayonnaise, low-fat
2	Tbsp	chives, dried
2	Tbsp	dill, dried
2	Tbsp	lemon juice

Mix all ingredients in bowl and refrigerate.

Makes 5 servings
Serving Size: 2 Tbsp
Per Serving:

Calories	39	Carbohydrate	4 g
Total Fat	2 g	Calcium	76 mg
Saturated Fat	0 g	Magnesium	10 mg
Cholesterol	3 mg	Potassium	110 mg
Sodium	66 mg	Fiber	0 g
Protein	2 g		

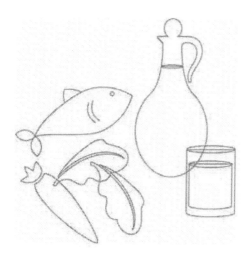

Day 6

Spicy Baked Fish

1	pound	salmon (or other fish) fillet
1	Tbsp	olive oil
1	tsp	spicy seasoning, salt-free

1. Preheat oven to 350 °F. Spray a casserole dish with cooking oil spray.
2. Wash and dry fish. Place in dish. Mix oil and seasoning and drizzle over fish.
3. Bake uncovered for 15 minutes or until fish flakes with fork. Cut into 4 pieces. Serve with rice.

Makes 4 servings
Serving Size: 1 piece (3 oz)
Per Serving:

Calories	192	Carbohydrate	<1 g
Total Fat	11 g	Calcium	18 mg
Saturated Fat	2 g	Magnesium	34 mg
Cholesterol	63 mg	Potassium	560 mg
Sodium	50 mg	Fiber	0 g
Protein	23 g		

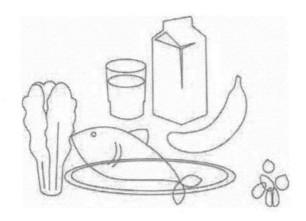

Day 6

Scallion Rice

4½	cups	cooked brown rice (cooked in unsalted water)
1½	tsp	bouillon granules, low sodium
¼	cup	scallions (green onions), chopped

1. Cook rice according to directions on the package.
2. Combine the cooked rice, scallions, and bouillon granules and mix well.
3. Measure 1-cup portions and serve.

Makes 5 servings
Serving Size: 1 cup
Per Serving:

Calories	200	Carbohydrate	41 g
Total Fat	2 g	Calcium	23 mg
Saturated Fat	0 g	Magnesium	77 mg
Cholesterol	0 mg	Potassium	92 mg
Sodium	18 mg	Fiber	6 g
Protein	5 g		

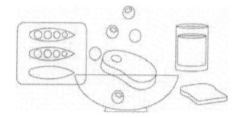

Day 7

Zucchini Lasagna

1/2	pound	cooked lasagna noodles, cooked in unsalted water
3/4	cup	part-skim mozzarella cheese, grated
1 1/2	cups	cottage cheese,* fat-free
1/4	cup	Parmesan cheese, grated
1 1/2	cups	raw zucchini, sliced
2 1/2	cups	low-sodium tomato sauce
2	tsp	basil, dried
2	tsp	oregano, dried
1/4	cup	onion, chopped
1	clove	garlic
1/8	tsp	black pepper

1. Preheat oven to 350 °F. Lightly spray a 9- by 13-inch baking dish with vegetable oil spray.
2. In a small bowl, combine 1/8 cup mozzarella and 1 Tbsp Parmesan cheese. Set aside.
3. In a medium bowl, combine remaining mozzarella and Parmesan cheese with all the cottage cheese. Mix well and set aside.
4. Combine tomato sauce with remaining ingredients. Spread a thin layer of tomato sauce in the bottom of the baking dish. Add a third of the noodles in a single layer. Spread half of the cottage cheese mixture on top. Add a layer of zucchini.
5. Repeat layering. Add a thin coating of sauce. Top with noodles, sauce, and reserved cheese mixture. Cover with aluminum foil.
6. Bake 30 to 40 minutes. Cool for 10 to 15 minutes. Cut into 6 portions.

Makes 6 servings
Serving Size: 1 piece
Per Serving:

Calories	200	Carbohydrate	24 g
Total Fat	5 g	Calcium	310 mg
Saturated Fat	3 g	Magnesium	46 mg
Cholesterol	12 mg	Potassium	593 mg
Sodium	368 mg	Fiber	3 g
Protein	15 g		

* To reduce sodium, use low-sodium cottage cheese. New sodium content for each serving is 165 mg.

To Learn More

NHLBI Health Information Center
P.O. Box 30105
Bethesda, MD 20824–0105
Phone: 301–592–8573
TTY: 240–629–3255
Fax: 301–592–8563

Provides information on the
prevention and treatment of heart
disease and offers publications
on heart health and heart disease.

NHLBI Heart Health
Information Line
1–800–575–WELL

Provides toll-free recorded messages.

Also, check out these online resources:

General Health Information
NHLBI Web site: www.nhlbi.nih.gov
DHHS Web site: www.healthfinder.gov
Diseases and Conditions A–Z Index:
www.nhlbi.nih.gov/health/dci/index/html

Your Guide To Better Health Series
Your Guide Homepage: http://hp2010.nhlbihin.net/yourguide featuring:
  Your Guide to Lowering High Blood Pressure With DASH
  Your Guide to Lowering Your Cholesterol With TLC
  Your Guide to Physical Activity

Nutrition
Dietary Guidelines for Americans 2005 and A Healthier You:
  www.healthierus.gov/dietaryguidelines/
How to Understand and Use the Nutrition Facts Label:
  www.cfsan.fda.gov/~dms/foodlab.html
MyPyramid and other nutrition information:
  www.mypyramid.gov and www.nutrition.gov

Physical Activity
The President's Council on Physical Fitness and Sports: www.fitness.gov
Exercise: A Guide from NIA:
  http://www.niapublications.org/exercisebook/exerciseguidecomplete.pdf

Weight

Aim for a Healthy Weight: http://healthyweight.nhlbi.nih.gov.

Menus and recipes were analyzed using the Minnesota Nutrition Data System software—Food Data Base version NDS-R 2005—developed by the Nutrition Coordinating Center, University of Minnesota, Minneapolis, MN.

Made in the USA
Middletown, DE
22 May 2018